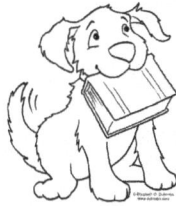

The Healing Power of Essential Oils
A Reference Guide

K. B. LeMere, ND

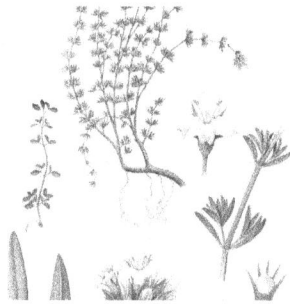

Health by Design Publishing

Dallas, Texas

I am blessed to have three loving men in my life:

My husband for the countless hours of time together he has given up,

My son for his encouragement to press on,

My father who taught me I can do anything through Christ that strengths me.

This book is dedicated to them.

The Healing Power of Essential Oils
A Reference Guide

Copyright © 2016

K. B. LeMere, ND

E-*book*

Health by Design Publishing

Dallas, Texas

Author Information

Email: drklemere@gmail.com

Web: http//www.author-kblemere.com

Book in Print

ISBN 9780983958185

9 780983 958185

Printed in the United States of America

Contents

History of Essential Oils

The healing powers of essential oils started with aromatherapy in ancient Egypt in the kingdom of Sheba, the "land of milk and honey". The use of aromatherapy dates back thousands of years. Egypt was a very prosperous country, which controlled the production of frankincense and myrrh. Egyptian priests developed a very sophisticated pharmacy, using large quantities of aromatics for the preparation and preservation of mummies. In addition, aromatics were refined into oils used by Cleopatra for skin care. Jasmine has a romantic reputation from Cleopatra who claimed it made Marc Antony fall in love with her.

For more than six thousand years, Egypt has been recognized as the birthplace of medicine, perfumery, and pharmacy. In 1989, Gary Young, a US citizen studying in France, brought lavender to the United States to start a lavender farm in Utah. He peaked such an interest in the farming community that it drew attention from holistic medical professionals. Using the knowledge he gained in Europe, Gary Young started traveling and speaking to professionals about the use of essential oils.

The Chinese may have been one of the first cultures to use aromatic plants for well-being. Their practices involved burning incense to help create harmony and balance, a form of aromatherapy.

Oils of cedar-wood, clove, cinnamon, nutmeg, and myrrh were used by the Egyptians to embalm the dead. They also used infused oils and herbal preparations for spiritual, medicinal, fragrant, and cosmetic use. It is thought that the Egyptians coined the term perfume, from the Latin *per fumum*, which translates as through the smoke.

Greek mythology credits the gift and knowledge of perfumes to the gods. The Greeks also recognized the medicinal and aromatic benefits of plants. Hippocrates, commonly called the "father of medicine" practiced fumigations for both aromatic and medicinal benefit. *Megaleion*, a Greek perfume, was created with myrrh in a fatty-oil base and used for its aroma, anti-inflammatory, and healing properties.

The distillation of essential oils came with the invention of a coiled cooling pipe in the 11th century. Avicenna, a Persian inventor, invented a coiled pipe, which allowed the plant vapor and steam to cool down more effectively.

In the 12 century, an Abbess of Germany named Hildegard grew and distilled lavender for its medicinal properties.

The 15th century brought more plants being distilled to create essential oils. *Paracelcus*, an alchemist medical doctor, is credited with coining the term Essence, and his studies challenged the nature of alchemy as he focused on plants as medicines.

During the earlier part of the 20th century, a French chemist by the name of *Rene Maurice Gattlefosse* became interested in the use of essential oils for their medicinal use.

Today many manufacturers produce essential oils. Caution must be taken when purchasing. Purity is the most important thing to recognize. Remember you get what you pay for.

The Method

Essential oils have three primary uses:

1. Aromatherapy, meaning to diffuse oil into the air for healing, or as an antiseptic to clean the air.
2. Applying oils for healing using massage techniques.
3. Applying specific oils to a specific organ or muscle for healing.

Aromatherapy is actually a word created by French chemist, Rene' Maurice Gattefosse, Ph.D, in 1920. Dr. Gattefosse determined that aromatic substances in many flowers, trees, shrubs, herbs, bushes, roots, seeds, leaves, stems, and flowering petals, contained healing properties in their semi-oily resin.

Essential oils have the ability in their chemical structure to penetrate the cell wall and transport oxygen and nutrients inside that cell. Being antioxidants, they are found to help increase oxygen, therefore, increasing cellular oxygen. When applied to the body by rubbing on the bottom of the feet, essential oils will travel throughout the body and affect every cell including the hair, within 20 minutes. The following shows how the

Vita Flex points (nerve endings) of the feet relate to the rest of the body. These are not to be confused with reflexology points, which are different.

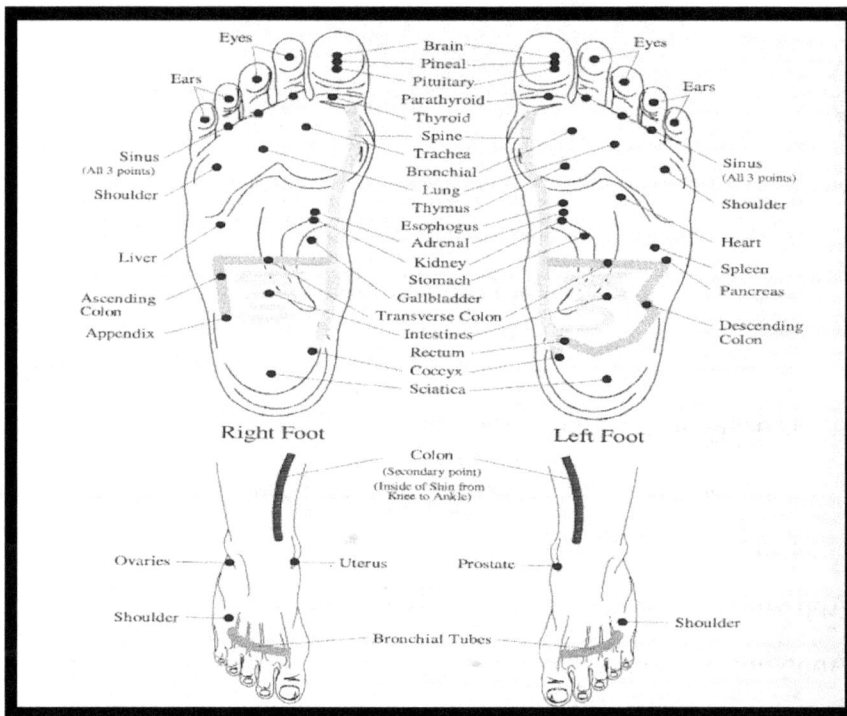

The bottom of the feet is always a place to start no matter what area you are treating. For example, if you are working on your liver, first apply the oils to the bottom of the feet, and then apply directly to your liver. If you don't know where your liver is located, we have also provided a chart of organs.

Energy and Frequencies

An energy frequency is described as a measurable rate of electrical energy that is constant between any two points. Everything has an electrical frequency. The highest form of herbal energy is essential oils.

We know that electrical frequencies are the driving energizing force in every cell. Each cell acts as a battery. Each cell has a different electrical charge on the inside. When a nerve cell is stimulated, a wave of depolarization travels down the nerve fiber. Potassium is released and sodium moves into the cell. When that current passes, the cell wall must re-establish the charge difference. A pump gets the potassium back inside the cell again. This battery sets up its own electromagnetic current. The collection of all these electrical forces, makes up about a trillions of our cells, constituting our energy system. The fatigue may be the batteries have run down. The cells need glucose and minerals for voltage potential in each cell. The body is a bioelectrical organism.

Essential oils frequencies penetrate the cellular biological level to strengthen the natural defenses of the body. The blood brain barrier is the barrier membrane between the circulating blood and the brain that prevents certain damaging substances from reaching brain tissue and cerebrospinal fluid. In June 1994 at the medical University of Berlin, it was documented that high levels of sesquiterpenes found in the essential oils of Frankincense and Sandalwood help increase the amount of oxygen in the limbic system of the brain. This is good news for Alzheimers, Lou Gehrig disease, Multiple Sclerosis, Parkinson, and Migraine headaches. The following shows how the Vita Flex points on the hands relate to the rest of the body. Do not confuse these with meridian points.

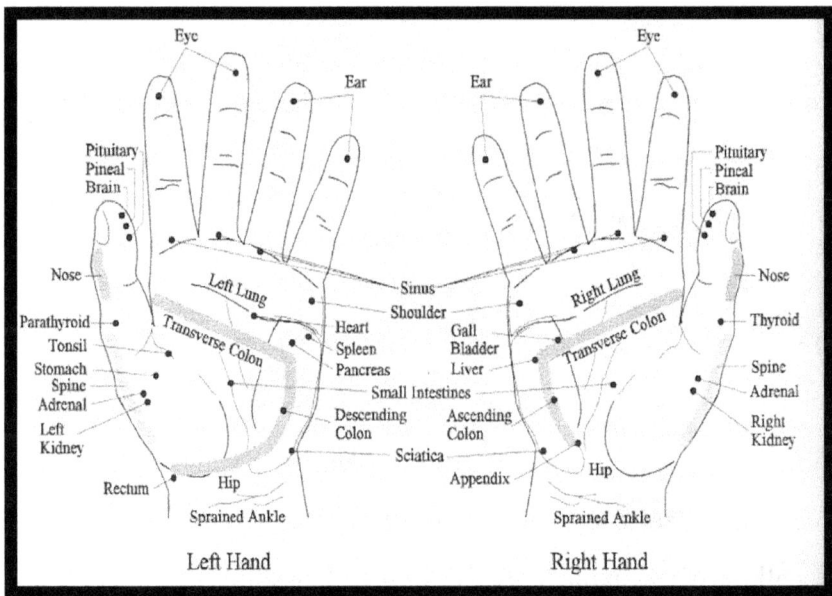

Eye — Ear — Ear — Eye

Pituitary / Pineal / Brain — Pituitary / Pineal / Brain

Nose — Left Lung — Sinus — Right Lung — Nose

Parathyroid — Transverse Colon — Shoulder — Thyroid

Heart — Gall Bladder

Tonsil — Spleen — Liver

Stomach — Pancreas — Spine

Spine — Small Intestines — Adrenal

Adrenal — Descending Colon — Ascending Colon

Left Kidney — Right Kidney

Sciatica

Rectum — Hip — Appendix — Hip

Sprained Ankle — Sprained Ankle

Left Hand — Right Hand

All essential oils are volatile oily substances that are highly concentrated extracts containing hormones, vitamins, antibiotics, and antiseptics. They have allopathic effects causing them to act like regular medicines. Other oils such as Bach flowers remedies or homeopathic preparations can have a more subtle effect psychologically. Certain oils have powerful antiseptic and antibiotic properties that are not dangerous for the body or skin. (A list will follow)

Oils are Agents of Plants

The method by which they work is miraculous. The oils are agents of the plant from which they come. Plants adapt to their environment; therefore, the oils use the adaptations from the plants' environment. When applied to the body, the oils carry information between the cells using the hormonal response of the plant. This controls the multiplication and renewal of cells, thus giving them healing effects on the human body. Here are just a few examples. A complete list will follow.

- Sage, traditionally known to regulate and promote menstruation, containing estrogen.
- Ginseng, a well-known tonic and aphrodisiac, contains substances similar to estrogen.
- Estrogen is found in parsley, hops, and licorice.
- Rosemary increases the secretion of bile and facilitates its excretion.
- Lavender, geranium, garlic, hyssop and sage all have healing effects
- Neroli, lavender, marjoram, rose, and ylang-ylang calm the effects of stress.
- Jasmine is uplifting oil for the treatment of depression or anxiety.

The Body's Sense of Smell

Odor molecules travel to the top of the nasal cavity fitting like puzzle pieces into specific receptor cells of the cilia. The cilia (see diagram) are little bundles of six to eight tiny hairs, which extend from olfactory nerve cells. These nerve cells make up a membrane known as the olfactory epithelium.

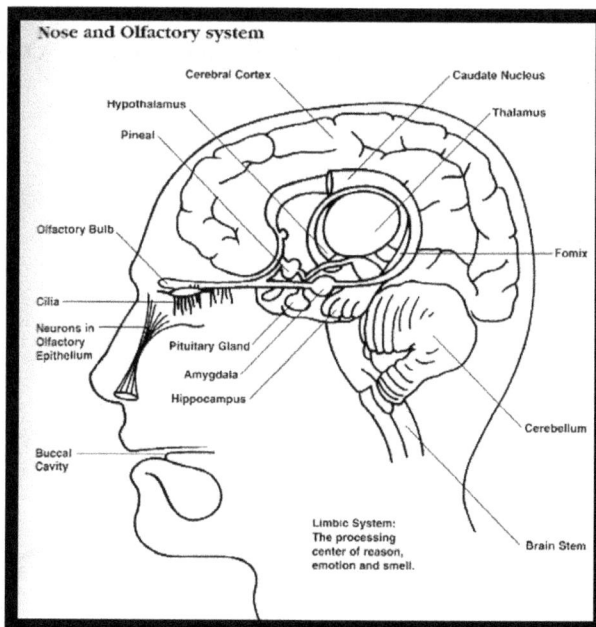

Nose and Olfactory system

Cerebral Cortex
Caudate Nucleus
Hypothalamus
Thalamus
Pineal
Olfactory Bulb
Fomix
Cilia
Neurons in Olfactory Epithelium
Pituitary Gland
Amygdala
Hippocampus
Cerebellum
Buccal Cavity
Limbic System: The processing center of reason, emotion and smell.
Brain Stem

The olfactory nerves respond to electrical signals and impulses and can remember smells. It logs all the information into olfactory memory. The sense of smell is very private and closely related to memories. Each individual's associations are different. The olfactory memories in the brain are very accurate and almost indelible. If you smell a certain kind of cookie, you think of your mother or grandmother baking in the kitchen, stimulating a memory of them. Therefore, essential oils can have some very profound physiological and psychological effects when inhaled.

Diffusion is one of the best methods of using essential oils, especially to clean germs from the air. For example: For an upper respiratory infection diffuse eucalyptus in the room, and apply a combination of oil over the lungs. Alternatively, for a sick room diffuse lavender, tangerine, or lemon. All have antiseptic properties.

Aromatherapy techniques use the therapeutic action of each essential oil to strengthen the organs and their functions, thereby acting on the defense mechanism of the body. It is important to understand the oils do not heal the body, but enable the body to heal itself without weakening the organs.

Application

Applying essential oils is very easy, but some precautions are necessary. Sensitive skin types are too reactive to apply directly on the skin, so here are some tips and ways to apply:

a. Compresses

b. Inhalation

c. Bath

d. Massage

e. Hand or Foot bath

f. Diffusion into the room

g. Warm and Cold compresses

h. Neat

Compresses: Compresses can be hot or cold, according to the condition. To make a hot compress, sprinkle 6 drops of essential oil into two quarts of water, as hot as you can bear. Place a small towel on top of the water to absorb the oils. Wring out the excess and place the towel over the area to be treated. Cover with a dry towel and a hot water bottle, add a third dry towel. Leave on 2 hours. This works really well for bronchitis. Another method is to rub the essential oil directly on the skin, cover it with plastic cling wrap, then a hot damp towel, and a dry towel. Leave on until the hot towel goes cold.

Cold compress is used exactly the same method but with icy cold water. Leave in place until it warms to body temperature.

Inhalations: The easier way of putting oil into the air is an aromatic diffuser. You can also use a vaporizer or humidifier, or just put 3 drops on a tissue or handkerchief and hold it close to your nose. Also, sprinkle a few drops onto a pillow to ease nasal congestion and to aid in sleep. Avoid steam inhalation if you have asthma. To use steam inhalation pour boiling water into a bowl and add 4 drops of oil. Inhale the vapors for 5 minutes. You can drape a towel over your head and the bowl to make a tent.

Baths: May be used as a single or blended. Shake 5 to 10 drops of neat essential oil into the tub while it is filling. You can also add 3-6 drops to your shower gel or washcloth.

Massage: The best healing method for essential oils is called Vita Flex. The oils are massaged into the feet using a type of reflexology. (See diagram in previous section)

Foot/Hand Bath: Sprinkle 5 to 6 drops of essential oil into a bowl of hot water, soak for 10 minutes

Air distillation: Use an oil burner or put a drop on a light bulb in the room. Always put oil on a cold bulb before turning on the light. Add to a sprayer and spray into the room.

Skin: Most oils applied directly onto the skin should feel soothing. If you feel a burning sensation, add some olive oil on top of the area. Next time mix the oil and olive oil together before applying to the area.

Beware

Before you purchase any oils from a retail store you need to beware of a few things! Over the counter mass manufactured oils are more than likely adulterated, not pure. Adulterated oils are processed with chemical additives and only parts of the herbs are used to make the oils. You can tell the difference by smelling each type. If you smell pure oil and then adulterated oil, you will know the difference immediately. You can buy the best from the originator, Gary Young online, at Young Living Oils. His fields are organic and the oils are 100% pure.

Beware that the use of essential oils may cause an emotional response. The sesquiterpenes, found in high levels in essential oils such as frankincense and sandalwood, help to increase the oxygen in the limbic system of the brain. This in turn "unlocks" the DNA and allows emotional baggage to be released from cellular memory. During the use of oils, you may experience emotions surfacing. If it is more than you feel you can handle, take a break from using that oil.

Try to identify you emotions by writing down your feelings. Go for a casual walk and think about what you are feeling. Talk to a friend. Do physical exercise to reduce intensity. Once you have identified the emotion try the oil again.

The charts on the following page show the essential oils and helpful uses. They begin alphabetically with single oils, followed by combinations.

Essential Oil Uses A-E

Single Oils	*Uses*
Basil or Basil Sweet	mental fatigue, rhinitis, spasm, snake bites
Bergamot	acne, boils, cold sores, eczema, depression
Birch, Sweet	arthritis, bones, joints, muscles, tendonitis
Brain Power	deep concentration, thinking clear
Cedar	bronchitis, anger, hair loss, diuretic
Cedarwood	acne, coughs, cystitis, hair loss
Chamomile (insomnia)	bruises, cuts, jumpy legs, scrapes, insomnia, teeth, acne, dermatitis, hair, menopause
Cinnamon, bark or leaf	infectious, viruses
Cistus	auto-immune, immune system
Clary Sage	cells, circulation, hemorrhoids
Clove or Clove Bud Redistilled	gums, teeth, digestion, appetite, colitis, bronchitis, dental, thyroid
Coriander	glucose levels, insulin, pancreas, sedative
Cypress	lymph, water retention, circulation, cellulite, edema
Dill	glucose, insulin, liver, pancreas, bronchial
Elemi	skin, glands, scars, muscles, wrinkles
Eucalyptus - Globules	lungs, sinuses and skin, expectorant, respiratory
Eucalyptus - dives	antibacterial
Eucalyptus - poly-bacteria	anti=infection, inflammatory, repellent
Eucalyptus - radiata	endometriosis, flea, sinuses, ear infection

Essential Oils F-L

Single Oils	Uses
Fennel	antispasmodic, cardio, respiratory
Fennel Sweet	digestion, stomach, intestines, kidney
Fir (bacteria air)	cold, cough, fever, flu, germs
Fir Needle, Canadian	bronchitis, respiratory, fatigue
Frankincense	depression, immune, mind, scars
Galbanum	body support
Geranium	hormonal, nerves, skin, tissue
Geranium, Egyptian	hormonal, nerves, skin, tissue
Ginger or Chinese Ginger	appetite, indigestion, throat
Grapefruit or white grapefruit	cellulite, obesity, water retention
Helichrysum	cholesterol, circulation, hearing, liver, phlebitis, scarring, skin, tissue
Hyssop	decongestant, toxins, lipids, scars, respiratory, mucolytic, parasitic
Joy	self love, joy to heart, romance
Three Wise Men	pineal to release deep trauma
Jasmine	cataract, cough, nervous, frigidity, absolute
Juniper	eczema, dermatitis, detox, kidney, acne
Juniper Berry Pure	nerves
Lavender	calming, cardio, headache, PMS, insomnia, sedative, skin
Lemon (purifies water)	air pure, water purifier, cellulite, lymph, kills bacteria, skin care, wrinkles
Lemongrass	digestive, sedative, tissue, vasodilator

Essential Oils M-R

Single Oils	Uses
Mandarin	digestive, liver, insomnia
Marjoram or Spanish marjoram	diuretic, headaches, nerves, spasm
Mountain Savory	body, immune, antifungal
Myrrh	athletes feet, bronchitis, coughs, decongestant, prostrate, diarrhea
Myrtle	cough, colds, thyroid, T.B.,ovaries
My Grain	all headaches
Neroli	digestive, mind, body
Nutmeg	adrenals, circulation, frigidity, gout, joints, muscles, nausea, nervous
Orange	mind, peace, mouth ulcer, skin, colds, constipation, flu, fluid retention
Oregano	metabolism, body, anti-fungal
Pain Away	arthritis, circulation, inflammation
Peace & Calming	Emotional
Peppermint	candida, fever, nausea, mental
Pennyroyal	kills flea's (danger to pregnancy)
Pine	opens respiratory system, bronchial tract
R.C.	respiratory, coughs, sinusitis, sore throat
Release	respiratory, coughs, sinusitis
Ravensara	herpes, muscles, nerves, viral
Rose; Moroccan, Bulgarian, Russian	asthma, cells, gums, sex disabilities, skin
Rosemary, Moroccan	memory, mood, sleep, blood flow, brain
Rosemary	dandruff, endocrine, immune
Rosewood	mental fatigue, skin

Essential Oils S - Z

Single Oil	Uses
Sage	hair loss, hat flashes, menopause, skin
Sage, Clary	hair loss, hat flashes, menopause
Sandalwood	cardio, lymph, pineal, pituitary
Sandalwood, East India	pituitary, oxygen, sciatica, skin
Spearmint	balance, burn fat, glandular, nerves
Spearmint, West Native	wt. Loss, glandular
Spruce	glandular, nerves, respiratory
Tangerine	calming, dizziness, nervous, sleep, anorexia, intestinal spasm, PMS
Tansy	bowel smooth, kidney, jaundice, stomach, sunburn, toothache, veins varicose
Tarragon	intestinal, PMS, sciatica, anorexia
Thieves	digestion urinary
Thyme or white thyme	cardio, fatigue, immune, weakness
Tea Tree, organic	antifungal
Valerian	tranquilizing, sleep, nervous
Valor	skeletal, physical alignment
Wintergreen	
Wormwood, natural	digestion, skin, liver and intestinal
White Angelica	memory, release negative, calming
Yarrow	indigestion, scars, healing of wounds
Ylang	heart, sexual disability, relax

Special Combo's

Combination Name	Uses
Anise Star	Emotional
Abundance	aura, emotional health, antiviral/fungal
Acceptance	overcome procrastination, denial
Aroma Life	cardiovascular, lymph, circulation
Aroma Siez	release muscles, relieve headaches
Awaken	reach one's highest potential, change
Christmas Spirit	joy, happiness, security
Citrus Fresh	right brain, creativity, joy, relax children
Clarity	mental alertness, trauma shock
Di-Tone	digestion, morning sickness, parasites
Dragon Time	PMS, cramping, irregular periods
Dream Catcher	enhance dreams, no negative dreams
EndoFlex	vitality, hormonal balance, metabolism
En-R-Gee	vitality, circulation, alertness
Envision	achieve goals, emotions, drive,
Exodus II	natural defense - immune system
Forgiveness	release negative memories, past barriers
Gathering	increase oxygen to pineal and pituitary
Gentle Baby	birthing process, reduce stress marks
Grounding	anchoring, awareness emotions
Harmony	stops allergy attacks

Special Combo's

Combination Name	Uses
Hope	move forward in life
Humility	emotions and feelings heal ourselves
ImmuPower	cold/flu, lupus, inner ear infections
Inner Child	reconnect w/inner child, abuse
Inspiration	bladder, kidney infections
Into The Future	leave past behind, move forward
JuvaFlex	liver & lymph detox, break addictions
Magnify Your Purpose	endocrine sys, creative, motivation
Melrose	clean cuts, rashes; fight infection
Mister	prostate, hormonal balance
Motivation	overcome fear, procrastination
Passion, Live With	depression, mood swings, loss of drive
Peace & Calming	relaxation, peace, sleep, depression, stress
Present Time	enpowering, forget past
Purification	cleans air, cuts, bites,
Raven	respiratory infections, T.B., asthma
Relieve It	anti-inflammatory, tissue pain, nerves
Sensation	arousing, skin problems
Surrender	aggression, stress, surrender control

Bach Flower Remedies

Dr. Edward Bach trained as a doctor in London. He was a highly successful
bacteriologist and later a homeopathic physician. After practicing and researching
traditional medicine for many years, he developed the belief that various patterns of
illness relate to certain personality types. This belief moved him to the discovery of
the flower remedies. The purpose was to harmonize the emotional imbalances that are
within certain personality types in order to counteract the negative, allowing healing.
The result of the flower remedies helped the person to change and bring them back to
a genuinely happy experience of life.

Developed through the work of homeopathy over fifty years ago were the Bach
Flower Remedies. The flower remedies are closer to homeopathy than anything else
is, therefore, training in the remedies involves understand how homeopathy works. If
you are not trained in medicine it is important that you understand the use of the
remedies are in conjunction with prescribed treatment and should not be used to
replace treatment. All healing processes involve both the mental and physical working
together.

Bach Flower Remedies are a holistic approach to health, disease, and healing. Dr.
Bach proved the first form of ill health begins with negative moods, and later

develops into physical illness. These moods are like a red warning light very clearly indicating an immediate need, otherwise serious illness will follow.

Traditional medicine does not confirm or deny that negative feelings affect the healing process. After completing a certification program at Harvard Medical School on natural remedies for psychiatric disorder, there is no doubt in my mind that negative moods affect physical healing and can actually bring on disease.

There are three beliefs that must take place to understand how Bach Flower Remedies work.

1. Diagnoses is based exclusively on states of disharmony in the person or negative feelings. Believing the flower remedies act directly harmonizing and healing.

2. Understanding there is no over dosage, no side effects, and no incompatibility with any other methods of treatment.

3. Usage of the Bach Remedies calls for no training in medicine or psychology. It does require a natural sensitivity with a keen perception of the other persons current mind set; therefore, using your ability to think and act according to their need.

The flowers are from certain plants that have a particular energy wavelength. Each plant-based quality is in tune with a certain frequency in the human energy field. For example, lets look at the negative feelings of hate and envy. This robs the body and organs of energy. The gland that is affected by hate and envy is the thymus. A patient with an under active thymus does not have an immune system that works properly. A healthy thymus is associated with love, joy, youth, and enthusiasm. There are three types of hate each using a different flower remedy:

General hate remedy is holly,

Festering resentment hate remedy is Willow

Hate that can see no redeeming features in others remedy is Beech.

Books and online training are at the Bach Flower Research organization at http://www.edwardbach.org. The Bach center can provide complete sets of stock remedy concentrates and published books plus other materials on the subject. Write to: The Bach Centre, Mount Vernon, Sotwell, Wallingford, Oxon, England OX10 OPZ

Warnings

Be aware of copies of the remedies or companies that claim to have the same product for sale. It is best to stick with the original source.

Bach Flower Charts

Bach Flower Remedies

Flower Remedy	Category	Negative	Positive
Agrimony	Over sensitive	Jovial, cheerful, love, peace. Are distressed by arguments, avoid by giving up, hide cares w/humor	Joyfulness and ability to confront others
Aspen	Fear	Vague unknown fears, for no reason, terrified that something is going to happen	Soul potentials of fearlessness overcoming and resurrection
Beech	Over-Care	Need to see good and beauty in all that surround them tolerant, lenient and understanding in all things	Soul qualities of sympathy and tolerance
Crab Apple	Despair	Things are not quite clean enough, despondent if treatment fails, cleaning purifies wounds of poison	Generous, little things will not upset composure, sees thing in perspective
Clematis (rescue)	No interest	Dreamy, drowsy, no interest in life, quiet people, not happy in circumstances, live in hope for happiness	Soul potential of creative idealism
Chicory	Over-Care	The needs of other, over-full of care, always finding Correcting and enjoy doing so, loved ones near them	Soul potentials of motherliness and self-love.
Cerato	Uncertainty	Not sufficient confidence in themselves to make their own decisions, constant seek advice	Principle of inner certainty, the inner voice, intuition.
Cherry Plum	Fear	Fear of the mind being over-strained, of doing fearful and dreaded things, impulse to do wrong	Principle of openness and composure
Chestnut Bud	No interest	Don't use observation and experience, long time to learn a lessons of daily life,	Soul potential of learning capacity and of materialization
Sweet Chestnut	Despair	Anguish seem unbearable, mind/body feels limit of endurance to give away, destruction left to face	Release, experience with God, able to believe, found oneself,
White Chestnut	No interest	Cannot prevent thoughts arguments they don't want from entering their minds, worry, mental torture	Tranquility and discernment
Red Chestnut	Fear	Difficult not to be anxious for other people. Ceased to worry about self, suffer and worry for those they love	Solicitude and love of one's neighbor powerful energy link between two individuals

		Doing good work, following calling, want to do for humanity. Periods of depression if task to difficult	Follows inner calling, above average gifts, natural leader, positive, responsible, confident
Elm	Despair		
Gorse	Uncertainty	Hopelessness, given up belief that more can be done for them, to please others try things but feel little hope	Hope
Gentian	Uncertainty	Easily discouraged, small delay in daily life cause doubt and disheartens	Faith, connected to God, also faith in the meaning of life, life principle or philosophy
Grape Vine	Over-Care	Capable, confident of ability, persuade others to do things as them, value in emergency	Authority and ability to carry conviction
Heather	Loneliness	Always seeking the companionship of anyone to discuss affairs, unhappy if alone,	Empathy and readiness to help
Hornbeam	Uncertainty	Not sufficient strength mentally or physically to carry burden of life, but they succeed in fulfilling task	Inner vitality and freshness of mind
Holly	Over sensitive	Thoughts of jealousy, envy, revenge, suspicion Self from no cause of unhappiness	Ideal human state, the goal we striving for in life. Love God, His beauty and goodness
Honeysuckle	No interest	Live in the past, ambitions which have not come true do not expect further happiness as have had	Capacity for change and ability to establish
Impatiens (rescue)	Loneliness	Quick in thought and action and wish all things to be done w/o hesitation or delay, work and think alone	Qualities of patience and gentleness
Larch	Despair	Don't feel good or capable as others, expect failure don't attempt to succeed	Self confidence
Mimulus	Fear	Fear of worldly things, everyday life, quietly bear their problems, do not freely speak to others	Courage and confidence
Oak	Despair	Brave people fighting against great difficulties without loss of hope or effort. Hate illness interfere w/helping	Strength and endurance
Olive	No interest	Suffer mentally or physically exhausted to no more strength, life hard work without pleasure	Regeneration, peace, restored balance, strength vitality, inner guidance, stress w/cheerfulness

Pine	Despair	Blame themselves, never content with their efforts or results, hard working, attach faults to self	Regret and forgiveness
Rock Rose	Fear	Emergency, appears no hope, sudden illness, frightened or terrified, fear to those around,	Courage and steadfastness
Rock Water (rescue)	Over-Care	Strict in way of living, deny self joys and pleasures want to be well, strong, active be an example	Adaptability and inner freedom
Star of Bethlehem	Despair	Great distress for a time producing unhappiness. The shock of bad news, loss of loved one, refuse comfort	Awakening and reorientation
Scleranthus	Uncertainty	Unable to decide between two things, quiet people, bear their difficulty alone, don't share with others	Poise and balance
Vervain	Over-Care	Fixed ideas confident they are right, strong rarely change, convert all around them to their views	Self discipline and restraint
Walnut	Over sensitive	Definite ideas and ambitions in life and are filling them Can be lead away from ideas, people pleaser	New beginnings, follows life goals despite adverse circumstances, not influenced by others
Willow	Despair	Suffered adversity or misfortune, have resentment in judging life, life in unjust, embittered, don't enjoy life	Personal responsibility and constructive thoughts, positive attitude, from victim to master
Wild Rose	No interest	Resigned to all that happens, glide through life, take it as it is, no effort to improve things and find joy	Devotion and inner motivation
Wild Mustard	No interest	Times of gloom, despair, thoughts hid the light and joy of life, no reason for attack, not happy or cheerful	Cheerfulness and serenity
Wild Oat	Uncertainty	Ambitions to do something of prominence in life, who enjoy all possible, life to the fullest, but no calling	Vocation and purposefulness

Water Violet	Loneliness	Like to be alone, quiet people, independent, capable self reliant, go their own way, clever, talented, calmness	Humility and wisdom
Wild Centaury	Over sensitive	Kind, quiet gentle, over-anxious to serve. Nature leads them to do more than their share. Neglects own life job	Qualities of self-determination and self-realization

Quick Tips

Stop Headaches and Migraines: Try this: place 3 drop of the essential oil My Grain (order from Young Living) into the palm of your hand, cup your hands over your nose and breathe only the oil for two to three minutes. You will have relief because the frequencies of this oil open up the constricted blood vessels in the brain allowing oxygen to flow, therefore, relieving the pain.

Stop Spreading Germs: Try this: use a diffuser in the room of the sick person and pick one of the oils that have antibacterial properties to diffuse. Oils such as: Basil, Bergamot, Cassia, Cedar wood, Chamomile, Citronella, citrus oils, Cinnamon, Clary Sage, Clove, Cypress, Eucalyptus, Fir, Geranium, Grapefruit, Juniper, Lavender, Lemon, Marjoram, Melaleuca, Mountain Savory Neroli, Oregano, Purification, Raven Sara, RC, Rosemary, Rosewood, Sacred Mountain, Spearmint, Tarragon, Thieves, Thyme, Wild Tansy.

Dishwater, Clothes Washers and Dryers: Add a couple drops of Melrose or Lemon to dishwater for clean dishes and a great smelling kitchen. Use Lemon or another citrus oil to take gum out of clothes. Purification in the wash water kills bacteria and germs in clothes or put a few drops on a cloth and place in the dryer.

Cleaning and Disinfecting: Put a few drops of Lemon, Spruce, or Fir oil on a dust cloth or 10 drops in water in spray bottle to polish furniture or to disinfect bathrooms and kitchen.

Remodeling or Painting: To remove paint fumes add one bottle (15-ml) of oil to a five-gallon bucket of paint. Stir vigorously.

Quick Tips for Pets

Our pets give us unconditional love and loyalty, and we should pay just as much attention to them. Almost any herbal treatment that is fit for human use can be used for your pets. Make sure to reduce the dosage to adjust for the difference in size. Give the herbs in capsule form.

LINIMENT FOR LEG STRAINS: Bring 1 quart of cider vinegar to gentle boil. Add 2 tablespoons of cayenne pepper and continue to gently boil for 10 minutes. Apply to the area needed twice daily. This increases stimulation to the area. It is good to use when treating horses for leg strains. It can also be applied to the chest area for congestion and colds.

RHEUMATISM: Put 6 drops of oil of rosemary in ½ cup of water. Use this to massage the area that needs pain relief. For older dogs take a pillow that your dog sleeps on and stuff it with dried male fern leaves. This not only alleviates pain for the dog, it will also discourage fleas.

STOP FLEAS: Give your dog 1 tablet of 100 mg thiamine daily. You can also add to their food.

DRY SHAMPOO FOR PETS: Split a vanilla bean and place it in 1 quart of orrisroot powder or cornmeal. Cover and let sit for 1 week. Sprinkle over the animal and brush it in thoroughly. Then brush it out.

MANGE: Mange is caused by mites. Humans can contract mange from their pets, but is known as scabies in humans. It is a communicable disease, so be sure to treat your pet at the first sign or mange. The symptoms are the loss of hair and itching. Mix 2 tablespoons each of garlic powder and goldenseal powder. Add to ¼ cup of olive oil. Apply frequently to affected area.

EYE WASH: Put 2 tablespoons of comfrey and 2 tablespoons bruised fennel seeds in 1 cup of water. Bring to a boil and remove from heat. Steep until cool. Keep refrigerated and use by putting in the eye with an eyedropper.

EAR CARE: Clean the ears of your pets by dipping a cotton swab in wormwood oil. This should prevent any problems with ear mites.

DOG FOOT PADS: Split an Aloe Vera leaf and rub on the pads of the dog's foot. Massage in thoroughly and reapply frequently.

Quick Tips for Gardening

ROSE CARE: Turnips and anise, planted around the roses, will discourage aphids and spider mites. Put tobacco in the blender and add water. Blend well and use this as a spray to control aphids. Put several cloves of garlic in the blender with water. Blend well and use a spray to control aphids.

INSECT OIL SPRAY: Mix together 1 cup of liquid detergent, ½ cup of fish oil and ½ cup of number 10 mineral oil. Add the oil mixture to 2 gallons of water in a steady small stream, stirring constantly. Pour into sprayer and you're ready to go to work. It's good to control aphids, eggs of coddling moths, fruit moths, cankerworms, scale, and many other sucking and chewing insects that bother your free trees.

FUNGAL SPORES: Put equal parts of clematis, corn leaves, and the outer papery shell of garlic in the blender. Add enough water to cover and blend at high speed. Strain and spray affected plants until the fungus goes away.

Quick Tips for the House

FRESH CUT FLOWERS LONGER: Add 2 tablespoons of lemon juice and 1 tablespoon of sugar to 1 quart of water.

MILDEW TREATMENT: Wash down the areas that are prone to mildew with a strong thyme tea. Steep 1 quart of thyme in 1 gallon of water for several days. Use to scrub down the area.

TOILET BOWL CLEANER: Drop 3 vitamin C capsules in the bowl and let sit overnight. Scrub with brush and stains are gone.

ROOM FRESHENER: To freshen the air while you vacuum, simply soak a cotton ball with your favorite scented oil and add to your vacuum cleaner bag.

FURNITURE POLISH: Add 1 tablespoon of lemon oil to 1 quart of mineral oil. Place in a spray bottle and use on wooden furniture. Rub in and wipe off

In Conclusion

Understanding the frequencies of the essential oils is not as important as using them to keep balance in your world. Remember not all oils can be ingested. Pay attention to the proper procedure for each oil, the location to apply it, and how to apply it. Make sure when mixing oils together you wear gloves.

Blessing of Health
drklemere@gmail.com
www.author-kblemere.com